Professional Traits of a Healthcare Leader

A Guide for Women Looking to Level Up in the World of Healthcare

Sonja Gunter

DH BOOK CONSULTING & PUBLISHING

McDonough, GA, U.S.A.

Professional Traits of a Healthcare Leader

Ordering Information:
Quantity sales. Special discounts are available on quantity purchases by corporations, associations, and others. For details, contact the author at the address above.

Cover Design by Mark Shan

Published by:
DH Book Consulting & Publishing
P.O. Box 3235
McDonough, GA 30253

www.dhbooksandpublishing.com

Printed in the United States of America

First Printing, 2020

ISBN 978-1-7334436-2-3

This book is dedicated to all the women whom I have had the privilege of coaching and mentoring over the years, the women who I currently lead and train to be leaders, and the women who are still discovering that a leader does indeed exist in them already.

Acknowledgments

I would like to first personally thank God for remembering me when I thought He had counted me out. This is my exodus!! To my children — my daughters Imani and Deja, and my son Aaron — thank you for being my absolute motivation to never stop pressing; I haven't yet. You are my very breath and heartbeat. I know there is greatness and leadership in you all.

To all the teachers in my life who taught me the word "assertive" when others labeled me as "aggressive", thank you for recognizing the leader in me from a very young age. Jeanne Pete, yes you. you had such a quiet impact on me when I moved to Atlanta. I find your strength and leadership inspiring. I wanted you to recognize the leader in me and when you did, it did something to me. You lit a fire in me that I didn't realize existed. Thank you for encouraging me the way you have.

To the fabulous Carlotta Eversley-Gabriele, thank you for your words of wisdom and for being so available to assist at such short notice.

To my best friend of thirty-five years, Christina L. Page, I know you and Michael have never stopped praying for me, and with me. I will never forget the day I called you, crying uncontrollably. Michael prayed like never before as you quietly wept and prayed in the background. I heard you my friend. Your prayers saved my life that day.

To everyone who has encouraged, motivated, inspired or even walked away from me, I sincerely thank you. For every lesson is a blessing and with each encounter I become a better person.
Last but not least, to my husband, John L. Gunter, thank you for allowing me space to stretch out and explore who I am as an individual. This speaks to how secure you are in being my husband and that you trust me as your wife. I really don't know a better person to live this journey with. Your calm is my refuge. It is our time... now.

Foreword

The first nursing revolution was sparked by one individual, Florence Nightingale. It was primarily to formalize and structure the nursing industry in which specific ideals of caring, compassion, nurture, and patience were the foundation for what became the core of nursing. There needs to be another revolution, this time spawn collectively with the purpose to restore the ideals of healthcare in general — back to practical application. When truth is used to evaluate the backdrop of how healthcare is currently — and for far too long, experienced — the ideals of what healthcare is supposed to be are practically non-existent.

With the Affordable Care Act sparking terms like "Patient Experience" to address the need to improve patient care and the quality of medicine applied, it's easy to get lost in the malaise of such a complexed document, or to lose the essence of what Florence Nightingale made and demonstrated that is actually simple. And with all the technological advances that continues to flood healthcare for utilization, the one constant element is too much and also too easily ignored. The "human element."

As a healthcare leader, we first must embody what we want to teach. Therefore, we must understand the dynamics of the group we are leading, identify what is missing in terms of character or behavior, and be able to convey our message clearly and concisely. Effecting change is first "being the change we want to see" as Ghandi so eloquently put it indicating that we have to first look at "the man in the mirror." What have we as leaders done wrong to bring us to where we are? Where did we go wrong? How could we have gone wrong with all the advancements we've made? Unfortunately, advancement often equals leaving behind, when advancement should mean extending. That which has been left behind, are the very simple notions that hold greater value than that which we believe are advancements in medicine; that is the basic ideals of what healthcare was founded on.

This book is not just a reminder of these ideals, but it relays the steps back to the practice of them. Schools focus on educating their students on theories of the human body, disease processes, and chemical interactions, but there is a significant depravity on these ideals. When studying what Florence Nightingale focused on and other pioneers in the healthcare industry, it was clearly on the intangible human traits that healthcare leaders hold a superior practice on; these caring and compassionate instincts is what made us leaders special.

Decades ago, before emotional intelligence became the newest popular psychological concept for self-help professions to hone on, the healthcare industry was already masters at exemplifying such traits.

This book not only re-introduces the ideals that built and revolutionized the healthcare industry, but it allows readers to tap into those innate human qualities that industry leaders possess that sets us apart from other professionals. This book will help you restore the passion that may have been extinguished by the fights and plights of trying to keep one's head above the heaves of health

care. This book reminds you that you can remain "Authentic" and maintain "Integrity" regardless of your environment.
I have never met a woman that went into this industry for any reason other than a passion for taking care of people. It is growingly harder to keep passion for healthcare alive in an industry where compassion is nearly dead. But if you are like me, who has struggled to keep the fire of what I love to do going, then reading this book may be exactly what the "Nurse" has ordered!

Carlotta Gabriele, MSN-Ed, RN
CEO of Elite Nursing Services
Clinical Professor
Healthcare Leader

Table of Contents

Introduction

A recent study in Harvard Business Review, concluded that women rated 84% higher in almost every leadership skill than men. (1) Women all over are taking lead in various industries and doing a great job. When it comes to healthcare, we are taking control of our health via breast cancer awareness, education and testing. We are learning more about cervical cancer and now know that the rate of death from cervical cancer has decreased significantly as a result of the increased use of pap testing. Although these are absolute reasons to celebrate, we are facing the grim truth that a lot of women are still on the verge of losing the access to this vital healthcare with the impending talks of the eradication of the Affordable Care Act.

This book is not about politics or to sway you to think a certain way, but a testament to the fact that we need more women in key leadership positions where true change can be enacted. In 2019, we are still finding a need to bring our issues to the forefront of healthcare via marches, sit-ins and boycotts. In as recent as 2019, laws and bills were passed that put restrictions on how and when a woman can handle her own body. No matter where you stand on the issues, the fact remains, women are still fighting an uphill battle to have total say in how we want and deserve to be handled in the healthcare realm.

We see women leaders in healthcare all around us — in clinical leadership positions especially. But we were sold on the thought that men made better leaders when it came to operations and processes. Throughout the preparation and execution of this book, and quite honestly throughout my life, whether intentionally or unintentionally, I have studied women leaders.

I can recall as a young girl in school, having teachers that led the classroom with grace and perseverance, attempting to shape our adolescent minds into critically thinking adults. I recall watching my Godmother, a First Lady in her church, serve her husband and Pastor, all while making him shine as he preached his sermons on Sunday morning. She would hold him down behind the scenes and then take a humble seat on the first row and "amen" and "preach Pastor" all Sunday morning long. I recall as a young adult, my very first job in healthcare. I was an administrative assistant to a woman who was the Executive Director for a skilled nursing facility and rehabilitation center right up the street from my home. I remember how big her personality was and how she commanded the room when she walked in. For as well-dressed, well-spoken and well put together as she was, she was that much respected… and she wore high heels every day and never had a hair out of place.

As I wrote this book, I read books written by other women leaders, some well-known, such as our former first lady, Mrs. Michelle Obama, who in her book Becoming, shared how she had to lead from her husband's proverbial "sidecar". Yet the impression she left on our hearts is timeless and just as worthy of recognition and acknowledgement as the President himself. I read a few books written by women right here in Atlanta that I have had the privilege of meeting; women who are leaders in their own right. Women like my friend, Talisia D. Rowell, who penned the book, What Good Can Come from You? This woman teaches and trains new hires at Delta airlines while also motivating and influencing young girls on stages all throughout the Atlanta area. I had the privilege of meeting and becoming friends with the beautiful Yvonne Joyce Dunkley, the woman who turned her breast cancer diagnosis into a platform to educate other women across the globe about early breast cancer detection. Not only does she share her story freely with others, she raises money and brings healthcare professionals from all walks, to provide screenings and education to those who may otherwise never get the necessary attention.

Being a leader in healthcare starts way before the actual job title. Being a leader in healthcare starts within you before you ever realize it. Being a leader is a mindset. Too often than not, we are doubtful of our abilities. We lack self-confidence because society has taught us that women should be soft and demure, and leadership is about strength — a masculine attribute. But consider this, as a woman, we take on various roles in life that have already prepared us for leadership. We manage homes as wives and mothers. In this world, we learn to manage our emotions so that we are heard with respect. Being a leader is not about a title but about being an influencer. We are constantly influencing our children and communities when we speak and by the way we move. Even if we have been the one to influence others to do something questionable, imagine the impact you can have if you influence others for good.

Being a leader in general, you must have vision and believe you can achieve what your mind's eye sees. When I became a teenage mother at the age of eighteen, I had not envisioned that for my life. However, I did not have a clear vision for how I did want my life to go. I allowed other people to tell me what they thought I should do, how I should look and what I should feel. Once I began to form a vision for myself, I held on tight and although my life took many turns, I never lost sight of my vision. The sooner I changed my circle of influencers, the more in tune to my path I became. If you think you can continue to associate with those that are not moving ahead and expect that you will be a shaker and a mover, you are setting yourself up for big disappointment. There's an old saying that says, "eagles don't fly with pigeons". You can think what you want, but I am a witness that until you get in the company of those that can fly higher than you, and at minimum, as high as you, you will always be pulled down by the weight of others. It is not only okay to outgrow your current circumstances, but it is vitally necessary. Never allow the shortsightedness of the naysayers to convince you that you are too much. You are never too much, you just may be too much for them to handle because they feel their inadequacies in your presence; their issue, not yours. As you ascend into a position of leadership in life, prepare for some to be disappointed or feel let down. Don't let that worry you. In my honest opinion, if you don't lose friends, your moves may not be big enough.

As we journey through this book together, I want you to really understand that these leadership traits will work for life in general. There are some very specific mentions that relate to healthcare, however as you read through these pages, you may find that you are already a leader. I know I have. I have not ascended to the level of leadership I even desire yet, but I'm on my way there. Let's go together as we work to change the face of healthcare. Enjoy.

Chapter 1

Education

Education is for improving the lives of others and for leaving your community and world better than you found it.
Marian Wright Edelman

I recall as a child, the long lectures my father insisted I sit through about the importance of a great education. He would even go as far to say that you can't just be good in life, you must be the best. I never quite understood why he preached and emphasized a good education so much until I got serious about my own career path as an adult. I must admit, I was always an intelligent kid — I just didn't take school seriously enough. As a matter of fact, as far back as I can remember, I was always told that I was aggressive, mouthy and sassy. I was later told by a mentor that I was not aggressive but assertive. He told me I wasn't mouthy and sassy, but opinionated and not afraid to speak up.

School always came easy to me when I applied myself. I prided myself on being an excellent test taker. It wasn't until I went to nursing school and almost flunked out three months into the program that I discovered I had better get serious. In nursing school, anything less than 75% was considered failing.

As healthcare professionals, we are expected to excel. There is always so much changing in the healthcare industry that in order to remain relevant, we must be in constant learning mode. We must be able to critically think and learn how to assess situations from more than one perspective. As a leader in healthcare, there will always be an opportunity to make executive decisions that will directly affect someone else. Keep in mind, healthcare is about helping others. Whether you decide to be a leader in a clinical area or a leader on the operations and policy side, you had better be well-versed and knowledgeable in your specific area and confident about what it is you are talking about. People are counting on you and they trust you. There is no way possible to be a leader in healthcare if you lack education. You will always be required to learn, to study, to stay abreast of new techniques, revised laws and the latest industry trends. In healthcare, you never stop learning. Ever. I found that as I grew in my career, I needed to go back to school for more credentials. I would find myself sitting in rooms with other women who had accomplished so much more than I had, and I would feel quite intimidated at their level of education. Although I may have had more experience and even better skill, I did not get the same respect because I didn't have the required credentials for the position.

Pursuing higher education is not just about gaining new knowledge and skillset to secure a job. Furthering your education, at any age, shows people that you have the perseverance, patience and maturity to stretch yourself beyond what is basic. Getting a high school diploma or GED is commendable indeed and should not be taken lightly. However, pursuing a higher education degree or a technical trade, lends a different outlook because it proves to the world that you have what it takes to push yourself to higher heights.

I chose to quote Marian Wright Edelman to begin this chapter because of her impressive educational achievements. She is an American activist who advocates for children's rights and president emerita and founder of the Children's Defense Fund. Mrs. Wright Edelman graduated as Valedictorian from Spelman College in Atlanta, GA and went on to receive her Juris Doctor in law from Yale Law School during a time in American history that was riddled with blatant prejudice and racism. Despite this she managed to not only get her post-secondary education but completed it at one of the top universities in the United States.

What exactly does education mean? One on of the definition of education that Merriam-Webster gives us is "knowledge". When we break down the word knowledge it simply means "to know". If you study the etymology of the word know, it means "to perceive or understand as fact or truth". With having this explanation of the word, is it possible to be educated without attending an actual college or university? Absolutely. Many times, in life the best education is from life itself. I recall watching a game show where a group of very successful entrepreneurs were put on a team to compete against successful college educated individuals in a series of group projects. By the end of the show, the projects were judged by everyday consumers and the winners were determined by how much money their product made, how much product they sold, etc. I must admit, the group of entrepreneurs ended up winning by the end of the show's season. However, in healthcare, it must be noted that you can obtain leadership roles quicker with a formal education. There are some roles where advanced credentials are needed and you will find yourself hitting a ceiling without them.

With all that said, do not let your lack of advanced education keep you from seeking opportunities for leadership where you currently are. Believe it or not, many of you have the many years of experience in certain areas and you are qualified for a leadership opportunity now. Again, just keep in mind, the more formal education you get in your field, the more respect you will receive, and you will discover the sky is the limit. As you peruse the pages of this book, I will share with you the many traits that a leader must possess in healthcare and if you have mastered these qualities or at minimum, made a concerted effort to hone these skills, you can find yourself leading others around you. You may discover you are already a leader and it is time to negotiate your position and your money.

Take a minute and write down your educational goals on the lines below. Remember to include the goals that you are closer to obtaining and those that are as big as your greatest dream. I will never tell anyone their dreams are too big to reach, but I also know what it is like to dream so big that the vision can be overwhelming. When this happens, there is a chance you may give up. Think of it like losing weight. You want to lose fifty pounds but if you consistently lose ten pounds a month, the small progress keeps you motivated and before you know it, you're at your goal weight.

GOALS:

Now that you have written your goals out, write down the steps you are going to take to reach them. Start with the most practical.

Chapter 2

Integrity

"Power is only actualized when word and deed have not parted company."
Hannah Arendt

This is a good one! Integrity is a noun. So, someone who is said to have integrity has IT and all the things that are synonymous with IT. A person who embodies good character and is upstanding, is someone who deserves to be a leader. Consider the person you desire to follow. Don't you want them to be truthful to you? What about fair, decent and sincere? I believe firmly that integrity is the backbone to the healthcare industry in general. So, a healthcare leader must have… IT.

When I interviewed for jobs, it seemed I was always asked the same question, "What do you look for in a leader?" After some thought, my answer was simple, "Honesty… integrity." In my mind, if you are dealing with someone who is honest and integral, surely this is someone I could trust to have my best interest. In the same token, what I desire from a leader, I want to exemplify that same behavior as a leader.

I believe it was Oprah who said , "Real integrity is doing the right thing, knowing that nobody's going to know whether you did it or not." As a leader, your superiors need to have assurance that they can trust you to be on task and to perform in the manner expected, whether they are there or not. If you feel you need to be micromanaged in order to get the job done, you are not ready for leadership. Leaders do not require anyone else to hold them accountable, they can do that themselves.

Recently I stumble onto an article about the passing of Dr. Shuping Wang. Dr. Wang was a doctor in the Chinese province of Henan. (3) Back in 1991, she worked at a plasma collection site that sold blood to government-ran blood banks in the area. During her time there, she discovered that some of the blood samples were tainted from poor collection practices and mishandling of blood products that were positive for Hepatitis C. When she brought her concerns to the powers that be, it was decided by the higher ups that improving practices was too costly and they would continue in the manner they always had. This did not satisfy Dr. Wang, so she took it to the Ministry of Health. When the Ministry of Health heard about what was happening, it was ordered that the blood banks improve their collection practices and all donors were expected to undergo Hepatitis C testing. Ultimately her integrity caused her to lose her job and she was transferred to a health bureau. It was at the health bureau in 1995, that Dr. Wang discovered another public health threat. She discovered a donor who had tested positive for HIV had sold blood in four different areas. Again, Dr. Wang blew the whistle to the dismay of her superiors. Dr. Wang's integrity was greater than her fear of

retaliation, it was greater than her own financial gains, and ultimately, it saved the lives of many. What type of integrity do you possess?
If you go back to school or have already been in school for ANY healthcare related career, you have studied integrity. You will learn or have learned words like beneficence, maleficence, justice, code of ethics, etc. All these words simply point back to integrity. These words keep the best interest of others in the forefront. There is no escaping this necessary character trait in healthcare and without it, you simply don't have what it takes to be a leader in healthcare. You may actually be better suited for politics. Just kidding — I digress.

I have had the pleasure of leading many individuals throughout my healthcare career. As a nurse for sixteen years, most of my positions came with some sort of leadership responsibilities attached. One thing I have always tried very hard to do with all my staff, was to treat everyone fairly and with decency and respect. One way I did that was to adhere to company policy and procedure… the black and white of any organization. If you do this, you won't risk playing favorites among your subordinates. Now, that's not to say that exceptions can't be made to the rules. As we all know, there are always exceptions to the rules. However, it should be best practice to always stick to the black and white of policy so that you are never looked upon as being unfair. Trust me, once you show any sign of favoritism, you will never be respected as a supervisor. I know this firsthand.

I can recall a time when I allowed a certain staff member of mine to become my close friend. I was in a position to enforce rules with this person but because we were friends, I found myself torn between what was right and what felt good; company policy and the friendship. When that time came to answer for a service failure that she was involved in, I wasn't sure how to respond so I took it upon myself to deflect the failure on someone else. The other person had a part in the failure, but the truth of the matter was that my "friend" was ultimately responsible. When you are a true leader, issues like this can cause you to lose sleep. This was many years ago and I have since rectified my behavior through a lot of self-awareness and self-evaluation. Too late though; I marred my reputation with the staff at that company. One thing you will learn in this industry; trust is a hard thing to ruin and even harder to regain.

Think about a time in your life when your integrity was called in to question:

Were you able to stand on good ground?
If so, what helped you? If not, what could you have done differently?
Have you had a supervisor behave unfairly? If so, how did that make you feel that your leader behaved this way?

Chapter 3

Professionalism

It's NOT the job you DO, It's HOW you DO the job
Anonymous

I have the pleasure of speaking with many employers in the industry and many do group interview. During the interview process, management will pose a series of random questions to the group. Random to them, but there are some that they ask every week. I am told by one employer, the very first question they always ask is to "Please define professionalism in your own words." They said they get a variety of answers, ranging from appearances to how one works with others. To be completely honest, there are many ways to define professionalism and it incorporates many different facets.

Think about when you go to the doctor or even speak to someone over the phone about your cell phone bill. When you leave the appointment or hang up the phone, what do you think about those encounters that were pleasant; the encounters where your questions are answered thoroughly? It's probably easier to think about the situations when you weren't treated right. You were left feeling and or telling others how "unprofessional" someone was or is. Remember? Think about when you go to the doctor or even speak to someone over the phone about your cell phone bill. When you leave the appointment or hang up the phone, what do you think about those encounters that were pleasant; the encounters where your questions are answered thoroughly? It's probably easier to think about the situations when you weren't treated right. You were left feeling and or telling others how "unprofessional" someone was or is. Remember?

In order to be a healthcare leader, your words, actions and look must match. You have no room to say one thing but show another. You will lose all credibility and you will never get people to buy into you and what you say. To be a professional, you must make people feel comfortable to rest in you and the things you are talking about. This again goes for any industry. However, healthcare is one of those industries that people rely heavily on the supposed expert, YOU.

I have had to remind staff and myself at times, that if you want to be taken seriously, you must appear to know what you are doing and doing it with patience and a smile. I added the patience and smile piece because you can be the best at what you do and what you know but if you have poor delivery, you will run the risk of being considered unprofessional. I have been in the presence of some of the best doctors who were very knowledgeable but lacked social skills and have lost patients. Don't lose your opportunity to lead people because you have lost the ability to be human.

I read something recently that talked about always putting your best forward, looking the part, and dressing the part because you never know who you might meet in the streets. When people see you, they do just that… SEE YOU. There is no opportunity for someone to experience your personality or intelligence when they see you while you are not putting your best foot forward. Our society is a very visual one. If we all are being transparent, we judge a lot based on what we see. It is not fair; I totally get it and I agree. However, it is still fact. With that said, I have been in positions where I know I personally read resumes and was completely turned off by nicknames and slang names used in the return email address. I have been known to go to social media and look someone up if something about their resume gave me pause. Being professional is all about making someone feel comfortable that you are who you say you are, and you can deliver what you said you can in a package that is clean and respectable.

Think about a time in your life when you labeled someone as professional. What were some of the positive words you used to describe the service they gave you that led you to believe they were professional?

Would you consider that person a leader in your eyes?
What qualities did they possess that you want for yourself; or if you believe you have those qualities, what can you do to improve on them?

Chapter 4

Passion

"Without passion, a person will have very little influence as a leader."
Michele Payn-Knoper

I love passion. When most people think about passion, they think about the emotion that is shared in a romantic relationship. However, passion is simply a longing or deep affection for anything or anyone in particular. Passion is the fire under you that causes you to stay up late nights and rise early in the morning. Just as passion is necessary for a relationship to thrive, it takes just as much passion to make your dreams thrive as well.

I hear people talk about being passionate about a particular issue or topic, yet they haven't studied the topic, have no clue who the top leaders are supporting or opposing the issues, haven't attended any conferences… you get the picture. Please refrain from saying you have a passion for something yet have no evidence to support your passion.

Think back to a time when you first discovered you had a major crush on a classmate. I remember quite well. We were in the third grade and he was my first real crush. I could not wait to get to school each day to see his pretty smile and sit next to him on the reading carpet. He would walk me home from school and even gave me one of his mother's pearl and diamond rings. Of course, I had to give that back when I showed my mom. But I remember the feeling in my stomach of excitement to get to school. Even when he was mean to me, which was hardly ever, I defended his ways. We remained friends through the years and I am still loosely connected to his sister and keep in touch with her via social media. That's the feeling healthcare leaders have to possess about what it is we do. Without that, you will find yourself complaining that the work is too hard and that the pay is not worth the work. But what and who are we doing the work for?

Have you ever wanted something so bad you sometimes lose sleep at night? Do you find yourself at work and daydreaming about your future goals and plans because it's all you can think about? When I wake up every morning and when I lay my head down at night, I am thinking of ways to "change the face of healthcare". That is my one desire. I eat, sleep and breath healthcare. I am always looking for industry-related organizations to join and other industry experts to network with. I spend a great deal of time looking to see how I can master another skill to add to my resume that will make me more credible to my future audience. Writing this book is an indication of my passion for healthcare. I want nothing more than to see dedicated and passionate individuals delve into this industry and enact change whether on a global stage or in the patient room of someone who is taking their last breath. If you desire something bad enough, you will stop at nothing to obtain it. That, my friend, is passion.

As a nurse, I am truly passionate about healthcare operations and policy. That burning passion encompasses everything that I am and believe. I am the person at high school graduations cheering extra loud and feeling a bit of pride when I hear students desiring to go into any form of healthcare. I support it and I support all those with a heart to serve people. It is this type of passion that is needed to be a leader in healthcare. The people you will ultimately serve need to feel the warmth of your heart. It is passion that will drive you to work long hours to help someone else succeed. When you have a bad day, it is passion that will send you back into battle. With that passion, I find myself wanting to further my education and surround myself with those that feel the same way I do. Passion drives a person to reach goals and without it, you will fall short.

What are some things in life you are passionate about?

What is the evidence of your passion? Besides you telling people what you are passionate about, how can one tell what your passions are?

The most powerful weapon on earth is the human soul on fire.
Field Marshall Ferdinand Foch

The quote above talks about the human soul being on fire. I chose this quote because it speaks to the power of the intensity of passion. You, and you alone are a leader to be reckoned with if you would just tap into the energy of your soul. Close your eyes for a moment and think about what sets your soul on fire. I assume all of you who picked this book up have some sort of interest in healthcare. However, when you think about what sets your soul on fire, is healthcare still the "thing"? I mean, outside of that special someone that makes you feel good inside, is it truly healthcare? The quote at the top, in and of itself, is powerful.

When you hear the word leader, another word that comes to mind is powerful. There are arguments about who the most powerful man is in the world is. One thing that is certain is that all the conversations are around leaders of various countries. Whether we agree with their policies or viewpoints, what cannot be argued is that they hold the most powerful position in government office. Therefore, it is so important that leaders have the characteristics necessary to make the best decisions for all the people involved.

Chapter 5

Emotional Intelligence

"Emotional Intelligence is the ability to simultaneously govern your head and your heart, so you remain human yet in control of any given situation."
Sonja Gunter

Emotional intelligence is a trait that has a few different parts to it. It is truly a fascinating concept that has earned its' presence in many Ted Talks and psychology studies recently. I will attempt to shed light on this topic. I will tell you for certain, if you struggle with any of the following areas, you lack emotional intelligence and you will fail at being a leader in healthcare.

First, I would like to define emotional intelligence for you. Emotional intelligence refers to the ability to identify and manage one's own emotions, as well as the emotions of others. Although ambiguous in the over arcing definition, there are five key concepts that assist in helping you determine if you have it, you lack it, or you need to work on it. The first concept for determining emotional intelligence is self-expression.

Self-expression is the ability to convey your message effectively to others with clarity and in the proper context of how you are feeling.

The importance of this is that if you can properly express yourself, you leave no room for someone else to misinterpret your message. As a leader in healthcare, you will be responsible for giving directions. Your 'no' means 'no' and your 'yes' means 'yes'. If the people you are leading are not receiving a clear message from you, you have a high potential of service failures and for others to pick up on your weak areas. Nothing ever comes from that but manipulation and mistrust from the very ones you are expected to lead.

This concept of self-expression includes nonverbal language and cues as well. For example, I advise staff all the time, never tell someone they do not know how to do something. Not that it is wrong to not know but imagine being on the receiving end of someone who claims to be a healthcare professional and they give signs as if they are insecure or unknowing. It makes the person receiving care a bit apprehensive and will cause them to then question every move you make. You have now just created a scenario in which you, the healthcare professional, has lost control of the situation. Not a good position to be in. I advise them you are to always smile, never let your voice waver or your eyes lower. Let the person you are caring for know that you need to step away to call your supervisor for clarity on a step in the procedure and then take your directions from that point. When you are alone with your supervisor, it is there you can express your concerns or uncertainty and if your leader is a good one, they will either dispel your fears or determine that the task is outside of your abilities and clean up the situation on your behalf.

Self-Perception

Self-perception is paramount for anyone looking to be a better person today than who they were yesterday. Without self-perception, there can be no personal, spiritual or emotional growth. Self-perception is the third eye that looks within. It is the ability to "see" yourself outside of yourself and gain an understanding of how others are perceiving you. It is sometimes tough to do because it may mean admitting some faults and accepting some hard truths about yourself. It is something you have done if you have ever been in a disagreement with someone and later, dissected the disagreement in your head, made an attempt to see things from the other person's perspective and then re-evaluate your part in the disagreement. At the end of that process, if you do it right, you should have been able to conclude that you had a part in the conflict and been able to come up with a better way to handle the situation. This piece of emotional intelligence takes a maturity that is only begotten by life experience, humility and a connection with a higher sense of self. This is what people mean when they say they want to vibrate on higher levels and dwell with people who do the same. Those who lack self-perception suffer from living a shallow existence and never connect with people beyond the surface. There is no way a person will learn to be an effective leader without learning how to vibrate higher.

As women, we are always told to bury our emotions, especially in positions of power. However, I believe we make better leaders for that very reason. We can tap into our emotions and take other people's thoughts and feelings into consideration. But again, it takes maturity and daily reflection to do that and be effective.

Interpersonal Skills

Do you get along well with others? Are you a team player? Do you can communicate well with your team? Are you able to convey true compassion and empathy for others? If you answered yes to the above questions, you have the basic interpersonal skills needed to become a successful leader. A leader has excellent interpersonal skills. This is when a person has mastered the ability to communicate well with others, verbally and nonverbally. A leader that is considered a great one, has learned how to get along with others and manage a group of different personalities well. This is the type of person that other people just seem to like. When you have developed good interpersonal skills, you are a team player, dependable, responsible and patient. You practice active listening.

Decision Making

In order to be considered emotionally intelligent, you must be able to make a sound and logical decision even in the most challenging times. As a leader in healthcare, you are counted on to protect the health of many people. Not only must you safeguard your patient's health, you must consider the patient's family and how one poor decision from you may destroy someone's complete faith in you and in the healthcare system as a whole. You may have to make decisions about medications or whether to perform a surgical procedure. You may have to determine if the actions of a single mother puts others in danger and there is a need to terminate. These are very tough, yet very real, scenarios that happen every day in healthcare; sometimes all on the same day. You don't get to take a day off from leadership.

Even in down times, you are depended on by staff to give your personal and professional thoughts on a tough situation and a decision is made from that point. Yes, it sounds like a lot of pressure but a leader with emotional intelligence is in tune just enough to the emotional part of a situation, yet able to make a decision that is considered best practice for all involved.

Stress Management

After all the decision-making and smiling — although you want to cry — that you have to do throughout the day, you must have a place to go, mentally and physically, to just let it all out. An article published in the U.S. National Library of Medicine National Institutes of Health in 2016, discusses the dangers of burnout amongst healthcare professionals and the effects it can have on patient outcome. (2) There were three aims and objectives for the case study: 1. To explore the association between well-being in health care professionals and patient safety; 2. To explore the association between burnout in health care professionals and patient safety; 3. To explore the studies that measure both well-being and burnout in relation to patient safety. Through various research, data analysis and surveys conducted it was determined that burnout and poor well-being are both, in most studies reviewed, associated with poorer patient safety and has significant implications for policymakers and management teams within healthcare settings. To deliver quality patient care, the care must first and foremost be safe. The findings from this review suggest that staff well-being may play an important role in patient safety. As the leader of the team, you will have a huge role in seeing that your staff does not suffer from burnout while seeing that you also work at finding stress relievers for yourself.

I have included an emotional intelligence assessment for you. Please take the time to see how you score and then answer the questions that follow.

The Quick Emotional Intelligence Self-Assessment*

Emotional intelligence (referred to as EQ) is your ability to be aware of, understand, and manage your emotions.

Why is EQ important? While intelligence (referred to as IQ) is important, success in life depends more on EQ. Take the following self-assessment to learn your EQ strengths!

Rank each statement as follows:

0 (Never) 1 (Rarely) 2 (Sometimes) 3 (Often) 4 (Always)

Self-Awareness **Total __________**	
0 1 2 3 4	My feelings are clear to me at any given moment.
0 1 2 3 4	Emotions play an important part in my life.
0 1 2 3 4	My moods impact the people around me.
0 1 2 3 4	I find it easy to put words to my feelings.
0 1 2 3 4	My moods are easily affected by external events.
0 1 2 3 4	I can easily sense when I'm going to be angry.

0 1 2 3 4	I readily tell others my true feel-ings.
0 1 2 3 4	I find it easy to describe my feel-ings.
0 1 2 3 4	Even when I'm upset, I'm aware of what's happening to me.
0 1 2 3 4	I am able to stand apart from my thoughts and feelings and examin them.

Self-Management **Total __________**	
0 1 2 3 4	I accept responsibility for my reactions.
0 1 2 3 4	I find it easy to make goals and stick with them.
0 1 2 3 4	I am an emotionally balanced person.
0 1 2 3 4	I am a very patient person.
0 1 2 3 4	I can accept critical comments from others without becoming angry.

0 1 2 3 4	I maintain my composure, even during stressful times.
0 1 2 3 4	If an issue does not affect me directly, I don't let it bother me.
0 1 2 3 4	I can restrain myself when I feel anger towards someone.
0 1 2 3 4	I control urges to overindulge in things that could damage my well-being.
0 1 2 3 4	I direct my energy into creative work or hobbies.

Social Awareness **Total** ________	
0 1 2 3 4	I consider the impact of my decisions on other people.
0 1 2 3 4	I can easily tell if people around me are becoming annoyed.
0 1 2 3 4	I sense it when a person's mood changes.
0 1 2 3 4	I can be supportive when giving bad news to others.
0 1 2 3 4	I am generally able to understand the way other people feel.

0 1 2 3 4	My friends can tell me intimate things about themselves.
0 1 2 3 4	It genuinely bothers me to see other people suffer.
0 1 2 3 4	I usually know when to speak and when to be silent.
0 1 2 3 4	I care what happens to other people.
0 1 2 3 4	I understand when people's plans change.

Social Skills **Total __________**	
0 1 2 3 4	I am able to show affection.
0 1 2 3 4	I am able to manage relationships well.
0 1 2 3 4	I find it easy to share my deep feelings with others.
0 1 2 3 4	I am good at motivating others.
0 1 2 3 4	I am a fairly cheerful person.
0 1 2 3 4	It is easy for me to make friends.

0 1 2 3 4	People tell me I am sociable and fun.
0 1 2 3 4	I like helping people.
0 1 2 3 4	Others can depend on me.
0 1 2 3 4	I am able to make someone else feel better if they are very upset.

EQ Strengths – *Mark your EQ total scores for each domain to assess your strengths and areas for improvement.*

Domain	Score
Emotional Awareness	0 2 4 6 8 10 12 14 16 18 20 22 24 26 28 30 32 34 36 38 40

Emotional Management	0 2 4 6 8 10 12 14 16 18 20 22 24 26 28 30 32 34 36 38 40
Social Awareness	0 2 4 6 8 10 12 14 16 18 20 22 24 26 28 30 32 34 36 38 40
Social Skills	0 2 4 6 8 10 12 14 16 18 20 22 24 26 28 30 32 34 36 38 40

Measure your effectiveness in each domain using the following key:

0 – 24	Area for enrichment: Many opportunities for attention and development
25 – 34	Effective functioning: Consider strengthening
35 – 40	Enhanced skills: EQ is an asset. Use as leverage to develop weaker areas.

*Quick Emotional Intelligence Assessment adapted for Caterpillar Inc. from a model by Paul Mohapel (paul.mohapel@shaw.ca) (4)

Caterpillar: Confidential Green

Now that you have more of an understanding of what emotional intelligence is and where you rank, are you surprised by your score?

What area would you like to improve in?

In the areas where you may be weak, what will you do to improve?

Chapter 6

Authenticity

"As hard as it is, owning who you are and knowing what you want is the only sure path to affirmation… I want women to know they can get out of any situation if they return to their core source of strength: themselves."
Ashley Graham

I struggled with this quite a bit as an overweight young girl who found out at the age of seventeen, that I was adopted; being authentic Unfortunately, this information was shared with me by a neighbor who was about eight years my senior and apparently had heard the rumors in the street. I had never been comfortable in my skin and I had made a lot of bad decisions that could have really derailed my life in a major way. I never felt that I fit in and I always felt a bit of a disconnect with other people. To be completely honest, I still feel that way at times. My life did not begin to improve until I learned how to truly love and appreciate who I am — quirks and all. When I finally learned how to love myself outside of everyone else's thoughts and opinions, it seemed as if everyone else finally took notice.

As women, we sometimes suffer in the leadership realm as we find ourselves competing with men for top positions. We are told that as women we need to be soft and behave according to a certain standard. We must be attractive, but shy away from sexy. We are reminded to be careful wearing certain colors as certain colors signify power and control. Well… you want to know the truth? Like the old people use to say, the squeaky wheel gets the oil.
In the world of healthcare leadership, the 'squeaky wheel' is you, and the 'oil' is your money, your recognition, your promotion and your due respect. I am a firm believer that it does not matter what your gender is when it comes to leading a group of people. Do not ever let anyone make you feel that you are not adequate because you are female.

Ashley Graham reminds us that in order to be truly validated and secure the type of outcome in life that you desire, you must be authentically you. It is in you — and you alone — that you will find what you need to succeed in this life and become the leader you desire to be. Ashley Graham is a curvy model that is dominating the fashion world despite not fitting the typical model type standard. She has declared her beauty and because she believed it, she made others believe it too. That is the beautiful thing about being your authentic self. When you fully acknowledge who you are and are aware of what makes you unique, you can embrace the confidence necessary to be the leader you desire.

*****

When I started out writing this book, I knew the concept I was going for, but I wanted the audience that I wanted to reach to be very clear. My publisher would remind me to consider my voice throughout this guide and speak to the those that I wanted to hear it. This is the same thing I want you to consider as you learn and develop your leadership style. What type of leader do you want to be and how do you become that leader and still stay true to who you are? Your authenticity.

I took a class in school that dealt with different leadership types. Let's take a look at a few of the most common. (5)

1. ***Laissez-Faire*** : This leader likes to allow the team to make the decisions. There is a sense of empowerment that is felt by the team and they may even feel like their voice is being heard and appreciated. Not a bad way to go necessarily but you must keep in mind that this style of leadership may give the impression that "anything goes" and the team may take advantage of you.
2. ***Autocratic:*** This leader is a bit of a controller. This type of leader likes to make all the final decisions without considering the thoughts of others. There are times when this type of leadership is necessary in situations that require an executive decision. However, if a person consistently leads in this manner, you run the risk of others feeling as if you have no regard for their feelings. As a result, you will quickly lose respect.
3. **Democratic:** The democratic leader is one who operates in the middle of the first two. This leader considers others but is comfortable and confident in making decisions for the whole team when necessary.

4. ***Charismatic:*** It has been said that Oprah Winfrey is the perfect example of this type of leadership style. This leader has a personality that people gravitate to. These leaders inspire and motivate others. This type of leadership could raise morale and foster overall team success.
5. ***Servant:*** I must mention the servant leader; especially in healthcare. It is so very important in healthcare that the success of the mission is focused on the efforts of the team and not on a particular person. In my opinion, the best leader has servant leadership qualities — not only in healthcare but in any profession. This leader understands that a team is only as strong as their weakest link; it takes everyone to put their best forward to make the outcome successful.

There are a few other leadership examples beyond what is mentioned above. Again, I listed the most popular that are relevant to a healthcare position. In all honesty, a great leader possesses the traits of all these leadership types and understands when, and in what setting, to execute each one. The key to executing successfully, is to first understand who you are and then, put in the work necessary to perfect your skills. There is only one you; she can lead and conquer in any setting.

"True leadership stems from individuality that is honestly and sometimes imperfectly expressed… leaders should strive for authenticity over perfection."
– Sheryl Sandberg, COO, Facebook

Chapter 7

Cultural Sensitivity

Unity, not uniformity, must be our aim. We attain unity only through variety. Differences must be integrated, not annihilated, not absorbed.
Mary Parker Follett

Today we live in a society that dictates how we think about certain topics, how we dress in certain settings and how we view others based on our own values, upbringings, personal experiences and biases. All the chapters in this book are important, however, I cannot express enough the impact that understanding culture plays a huge role in how great a leader you will be and how well you will be not only perceived but received.

I have personally had the privilege of being born and raised in culturally diverse San Diego California. All of my primary education took place in the San Diego City School District and furthermore, I attended the School of Creative and Performing Arts from grades 4-12. At that school alone, I interacted with different people from all different walks of life; it became a part of my normal day to day experience. We had dancers, visual artists, performance artists, aspiring actors and actresses, musicians and everything and everyone in between. I must be honest and share with you that I wish I would have taken more advantage of the diversity in my formative years. I was exposed to some of the most talented people that have even now entered into the Hollywood movie industry and performed with dance greats like Alvin Ailey. In my neighborhood were interracial couples, Hispanic and Asian families, African American families, you name it, we all lived and played together on the same street.

After graduating and moving away from San Diego at the age of twenty-three, I ended up moving to the Midwest and lived there for sixteen years and now, I have been living in the southeast region for the past five and a half years. The invaluable and intangible life lessons I have learned once I opened my mind up to the beauty in the differences of others, have served me immensely in my climb up the leadership ladder in healthcare.

You must understand, in healthcare there must be a level of empathy that resides in all of us; whether your career takes you into operations or beside the bedside. I always question those in healthcare leadership positions who have never had to walk in the shoes — in some shape, form or fashion — of those they are called to make decisions for that will impact who they are and their quality of life. But how is that empathy developed? How does one go about learning how to be empathetic to others? You learn that by making a conscious decision to study and listen to others from various cultures and make an effort to discover why certain groups of people behave a certain way.

Before we can truly address cultural sensitivity, let's define culture. According to an article published by Livescience in 2017, culture is the characteristics and knowledge of a particular group of people, encompassing language, religion, cuisine, social habits, music and arts. In order to effectively lead a group of people, one must be sensitive to the different cultures represented in your organization.

I have the honor of serving some of the best staff I have ever worked with at my current place of employment. Although we all reside in Atlanta, we all come from different walks of life. A good bit of us are not originally from Atlanta but have migrated here from various parts of the country and a few from different countries all together. Understanding that, I must be sensitive to not offend and create rules or policies that may inhibit staff from feeling comfortable to come to work and yet still honor their culture. I believe we make a grave mistake when we try to impose our own social beliefs and traditions on someone else. We no longer make them feel like they are part of a team. As a result, we ostracize people which can cause division, a breakdown of the overall team production and the care of the very people we are there to serve. Cultural sensitivity is the state of being aware of the existence of the cultural differences or similarities between each other without considering any culture as a measure of something good or bad, positive or negative. Being aware of another person's culture creates a feeling of safety and belonging. When people feel secure and free to be who they are, lines of communication are opened up.

As a leader in healthcare, I have a serious problem when I see or hear people being ridiculed for thinking differently as if the way one group of people thinks is the only way to go. That type of attitude can create a hostile work environment and leads to poor morale.

We, especially women, have a great deal of stress that we attempt to cope with everyday only to come into the workplace and have to face the ignorance of the people we work with. Some days, if not most, we struggle to get out of bed to come to work, after having to manage our children, our homes and other outside obligations. Many of us work multiple jobs just to make ends meet, yet we come in and try to muster a smile through the tears.
If you think you have what it takes to be a leader in healthcare, it is imperative you learn to embrace all the people you serve; not just the ones who look and think like you. What a boring place this world would be if we were all the same. The funny thing is, if you take the time to ask questions and learn who someone really is, you will find out we are all actually more alike than we are different.

If you want to be a leader in healthcare, start by going into your job tomorrow and finding out something new from someone you work with. You will be amazed how that will make the other person know that you care, and you will be even more amazed to find out that you have the capacity to care more. Good leaders respect culture; great leaders change the culture.

Chapter 8

Social Media Networking

"I've always believed that one woman's success can only help another woman's success."

— Gloria Vanderbilt

I would be remiss if I didn't cover this subject. As women we know we can hold the keys to great information but not want to share it. There seems to be a fear among women that there is not enough success to go around. However, when one woman makes it, it opens the door for another woman to come in. We should only be competing with ourselves, not with others.

This is a subject that is so important in this age of technology and one that is not discussed enough in leadership conferences and professional gatherings; the power of social media networking and networking in general. I spend a lot of time on social media; some may argue too much. However, it's not just the time spent, it's the connections I make and the relevancy of my what my time is focused on, that makes me successful. I have just over 3500 friends and counting currently on my Facebook page. I promise you; I don't know half of them. Out of the 3500 connections, there are probably only about 125-150 people that I can say I have had some sort of personal dealings with; whether family or friend. The rest are people that have reached out to me, or I reached out to them, because we recognized there was a potential to network for business purposes.

Social media networking and networking in general has many positive benefits when used appropriately. I have literally been offered jobs from my professional social media page on LinkedIn. I was sitting at home one day looking for employment and received a message that a reputable company wanted to interview me. Within forty-eight hours of receiving that message, I was offered a fulltime position in a management role. The first impression was my social media page. By the time they met me in person, they had already formed an opinion of me.

I cannot express to you the many business resources I have come across that have had a positive impact on my career portfolio. And let me be clear, some connections do not bring immediate monetary benefit, but they all should offer some sort of insight you can use that may potentially lead to an increase in your bank account. When I served as president of Women Entrepreneurs of America Missouri Chapter back in 2013, I held a networking event that brought women business owners together to showcase their businesses and at the same time, raised awareness and money for a national charity. The day of the event, I had a phone conversation with my brother, and he shared with me, "The most powerful person in the room is the person who can bring people in the room." I didn't exactly understand what he meant then, but I understand it now. He was speaking to the power of networking.

Unfortunately for many, there can be detrimental effects on one's personal and professional lives if social media is not used in a responsible manner. I personally will look up an applicant on various social media platforms if I have any sort of uneasiness about their potential. While I understand that someone's social media page does not necessarily speak to their healthcare skills, it does speak to their character, discernment and judgement. Your social media page talks for you. You never know whose desk your name may come across, so you never know who's vetting you. It is so sad when I see young women with such great potential never get to the levels they deserve because the executive who is considering them has come across their page and found there is an image they do not want to associate the business, or even themselves, with. When people pull up your social media right now, do you appear to be an asset or a liability? Your social media is your personal brand. What message is your brand sending?

As a woman who prides herself on professionalism, I make it a habit to never post anything that will put me in an unfavorable light. I am very intentional about where I go and the types of people I associate with, so that if by chance I do appear in someone else's social media post, it won't tarnish my reputation or my credibility. First impressions are no longer only in person. Social media gives a very public eye into the personal lives of all of us. Many potential employers, or people who can introduce you to people who can quickly move you into places you couldn't get to on your own, have formed an opinion of you from your digital thumbprint. I cannot begin to tell you how many opportunities have been afforded me simply through leveraging my social media networking skills.

In today's world, there is such an "anything goes" type attitude. I am all for women living their lives to the fullest and recording memories along the way. However, we must consider what is good for now and what is good for the future. There are countless stories about people who have lost jobs due to something they posted on Facebook that they thought would never be seen by anyone outside of their network. There is a nurse right now in the news who did a video that many considered off-color in its humor and she is being investigated by her employer. By the time this book is printed, I can almost bet she will be without a job.

Being a leader carries a lot of weight. I am not saying you cannot let your hair down, but there is a time, place and audience that certain behaviors are appropriate for and social media is not it. Do not be afraid to re-evaluate your friend's list from time to time. If you find that the people you associate are offering you no value in terms of advancing your career or causing you to think about your future goals, it might be time to block or unfriend and start over.

Chapter 9

Reflection

As you reflect on your journey to leadership, I want you to consider a few things. Being a leader takes diligence and persistence. Leadership is not for the faint. When you are a leader, you literally have a proverbial target on your back. Although there are many rewards to empowering and motivating others to be great, there will be moments when you must correct and sometimes sever professional ties. There is no greater feeling than when you know you've made a positive difference in someone's life. When I hear young ladies in the industry tell me they pursued higher education because of something I did or said, I can't help but smile. Too often we, women, allow our struggles to dictate how our lives will play out. We are so many things for so many people, yet we neglect finding out how to get to our own finish line. It is time out for letting other people dictate our lives and tell us who we are supposed to be. The same skills you exhibit when you manage your home are the same skills needed to lead on your job. If you have children, the same way you handle sibling discords, are the same techniques needed for conflict management with your staff. The way we pick and choose how to face a disagreement with a spouse or romantic partner, is the same way we approach confrontation in the boardroom. The only difference in leadership at home and leadership in healthcare is the specialty of the healthcare field.

I have always said that I wanted to change the face of healthcare. I used to think that meant that I had to sit at the head of the table in a top-level administrative position. Then at one time, I wanted to open a school to teach people how to become Certified Nurse Assistants. I felt that if I could catch enough CNA's as they entered the healthcare field, that I could instill things in them that would encourage them to give better care and take pride in taking the first step in building their career. Then it occurred to me, if I wanted to change the face of healthcare, I needed to help shape up-and-coming leaders. I need to reach them on a larger scale.

Bibliography

1. Folkman, Jack ZengerJoseph. "Research: Women Score Higher Than Men in Most Leadership Skills." Harvard Business Review, December 10, 2019. https://hbr.org/2019/06/research-women-score-higher-than-men-in-most-leadership-skills.
2. Hall LH, Johnson J, Watt I, Tsipa A, O'Connor DB. Healthcare Staff Wellbeing, Burnout, and Patient Safety: A Systematic Review. PLoS One. 2016;11(7): e0159015. Published 2016 Jul 8. doi: 10.1371/journal.pone.0159015
3. Busby, Mattha. "Chinese Contaminated Blood Whistleblower Dies in US." The Guardian. Guardian News and Media, September 26, 2019.

https://www.theguardian.com/world/2019/sep/26/contaminated-blood-whistleblower-dies-in-us.

4. *Quick Emotional Intelligence Assessment adapted for Caterpillar Inc. from a model by Paul Mohapel (paul.mohapel@shaw.ca)

5. Themba, Chere, Grace Oshun, Shafaq, Lawal Samson, Pamela, Ayodele Aguisto, et al. "12 Different Types of Leadership Styles." WiseToast, July 2, 2019. https://wisetoast.com/types-of-leadership-styles/.

About the Author

Sonja Gunter is a Licensed Practical Nurse who relocated to Atlanta GA in 2014, after serving as President of the Women's Entrepreneurs of America, Missouri chapter, where she brought women business owners together for networking events and community meetings.

Since moving to Atlanta, Sonja has served several nonprofit organizations in various capacities. She has had the privilege of serving as Mistress of Ceremony for several events, the host for an awards ceremony celebrating women on a mission, keynote speaker for a CNA graduation, and recently sponsored and presented the Health and Wellness Award for the 8th Annual R.I.C.E (Rising In Community Excellence) Awards in Atlanta GA.

Sonja is a former radio show host and creator, which aired on Atlanta's newest and hottest internet radio station, mixx106radio.com. Sonja's years in nursing, her passion for helping others and her gift of public speaking, has created a platform that has given her an opportunity to provide education and resources on health-related matters to the communities that need it most. Sonja also uses this platform to uplift and empower women from all walks of life, especially those who suffer with self-identity issues due to her own experience with adoption and foster care.

Sonja is currently pursuing her degree in Healthcare Management. She is the proud mother of three biological children and many others she has been blessed to raise.

Thank you for taking the time to read this book. Find out more about the author at:

www.sonjagunter.org

On social media at:

Facebook: @mrsgunter2020

Instagram: sonja_gunter_2020

Made in the USA
Monee, IL
04 November 2026

67385889R10039